THE CARNIVORE DIET RECIPES COOKBOOK FOR WOMEN OVER 60

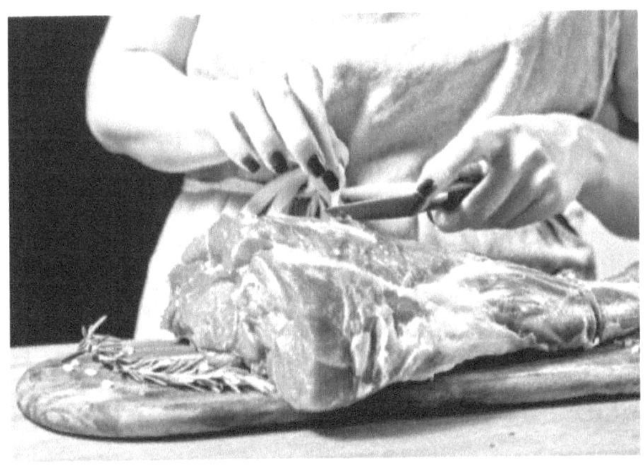

Discover The Carnivore Diet For Women In Their Golden Years, Rejuvenate Your Well-Being And Reclaim Your Vitality

Kathleen Scribner

TABLE OF CONTENTS

INTRODUCTION

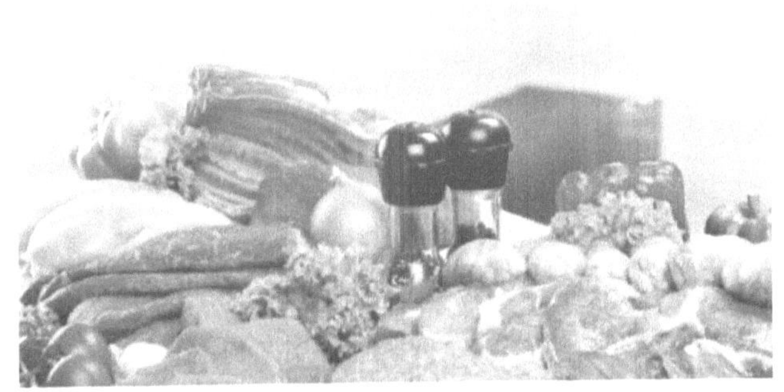

"**W**elcome to the Carnivore Diet, where the fundamentals of health correspond with our ancestors' most primitive desires. This dietary strategy, which is founded on a concept of simplicity, advocates just eating animal products (meat, fish, and other animal products) and avoids plant-based meals. Proponents of the Carnivore Diet point to a number of possible advantages, including better mental and physical performance as well as better digestion. Inside these dietary restrictions is a journey that questions accepted nutritional standards and allows you to investigate the significant effects of an animal-focused diet."

Benefits of the Carnivore Diet

Though results may vary, the Carnivore Diet is thought to have some possible advantages:

1. Simplicity: Supporters value this diet's simplicity since it minimizes the hassles of meal preparation by concentrating only on animal-based items.

2. Digestive Health: When adhering to a carnivorous diet, some individuals report improvements in digestive difficulties such as bloating, gas, and symptoms of irritable bowel syndrome (IBS).

3. Mental Clarity: Some advocates point to the diet's advantages for better attention and less brain fog, claiming an improvement in mental clarity.

4. Weight Management: Because of the Carnivore Diet's low carbohydrate consumption and possible

modifications to metabolic function, some people
have lost weight on it.

5. Possible Inflammation Reduction: Although
there is little scientific proof to support this, there
are anecdotal accounts of decreased inflammation in
illnesses like arthritis.

6. **Athletic Performance:** More study is required to
substantiate the claims made by some sportsmen
about improved performance and recuperation.

It's important to remember, however, that the
scientific community is still debating and
researching the long-term impacts and possible
hazards of the carnivore diet, such as nutritional
deficiencies brought on by the diet's absence of
plant-based foods. A healthcare provider should
always be consulted before making big dietary
changes.

How This Book Can Help You

For anyone starting a path toward improved health,
like Helen, a robust lady in her 60s, this Carnivore
Diet Cookbook is a beacon of hope. Helen found

relief from her erratic energy levels and intestinal problems after years of trying the stricter Carnivore Diet. But getting used to this new eating style was a difficult undertaking. The book turned into her friend, providing her with a thorough road map in addition to recipes. Its assortment of flavorful, nutrient-dense recipes enabled her to transition to a new diet with ease. From recipes for tender steaks to delectable seafood, every page served as evidence of how this diet might be both fun and sustainable. With its wide range of tasty recipes and enlightening advice, the cookbook became Helen's reliable guide, helping her rediscover her energy and a feeling of well-being she hadn't felt in years. It changed the way she saw food and gave her the confidence to choose a lifestyle that revitalized her body and soul.

CHAPTER 1

GETTING STARTED WITH THE CARNIVORE DIET

Understanding the Basics of the Carnivore Diet

The Carnivore Diet is a dietary theory that emphasizes exclusivity and simplicity. Fundamentally, this dietary strategy promotes eating meals derived from animals while avoiding those derived from plants. It includes eggs, meat, fish, and certain dairy products but not grains, legumes, fruits, vegetables, or processed meals. The tenet of the theory is based on the idea that our bodies are designed to consume a large amount of animal products, as our ancient diets did. Proponents of the Carnivore Diet contend that by removing potentially inflammatory or allergic plant-based ingredients, the body may be reset, possibly relieving symptoms including autoimmune disorders, energy swings, and digestive discomfort. Even if it's straightforward, obtaining premium animal products is crucial to ensuring a diet rich in nutrients. It is necessary to acknowledge this diet's departure from conventional dietary guidelines in order to comprehend its possible advantages as well as the current discussions among scientists about its long-term viability and health effects.

Preparing Your Kitchen for Carnivore Cooking

Changing your emphasis and ingredient selection is necessary to get your kitchen ready for Carnivore cooking. Here's how to arrange your kitchen:

1. **Stock Up on Quality Animal Products**: Invest in high-quality meats, fish, eggs, and dairy from trusted sources. Opt for grass-fed beef, pasture-raised poultry, wild-caught fish, and organic eggs whenever possible to ensure nutrient density.

2. **Eliminate Plant-Based Foods**: Remove grains, legumes, fruits, and vegetables from your pantry

and refrigerator to avoid temptation and make space for carnivorous staples.

3. Invest in Cooking Tools: Gather essential kitchen tools like a good quality meat thermometer, cast-iron skillet, grill, and roasting pans to prepare a variety of meat-based dishes.

4. Explore Different Cuts and Varieties: Familiarize yourself with various cuts of meat and different animal products. Experiment with organ meats, bone broth, and different types of seafood to diversify your nutrient intake.

5. Consider Seasonings and Condiments:bWhile the Carnivore Diet focuses on animal-based foods, some individuals include seasonings like salt, pepper, and herbs for flavor. Ensure these fit within your dietary guidelines.

6. Learn Cooking Techniques: Explore various cooking methods such as grilling, roasting, and slow cooking to prepare meats to your preferred level of doneness and taste.

7. Stay Informed: Continuously educate yourself on the nutritional aspects of the Carnivore Diet to ensure you maintain a balanced approach and meet your body's needs.

Organizing your kitchen according to Carnivore principles and putting high-quality animal products and essential equipment there will help you prepare tasty and filling carnivorous meals.

Tips for a Smooth Transition

Making the switch to the Carnivore Diet may be a big adjustment, particularly for women who are over 60. Using a Carnivore Diet Cookbook, here are some pointers to help you during this transition:

1. **Gradual Transition**: Start by gradually reducing plant-based foods while incorporating more animal-based options. The cookbook can guide you through this process, offering recipes that gradually phase out non-animal products.

2. **Consultation**: Before starting any new diet, especially one as distinct as the Carnivore Diet, consulting a healthcare professional or a nutritionist is crucial. They can provide personalized advice based on your health history and dietary needs.

3. **Experiment with Variety:** The cookbook likely offers a variety of meat, fish, and other animal-based recipes. Experiment with different

cuts, types of meat, and cooking methods to keep your meals interesting and diverse.

4. **Monitor Your Body's Response**: Pay close attention to how your body responds to the transition. Note any changes in energy levels, digestion, or overall well-being. The cookbook may offer insights into managing these adjustments.

5. Stay Hydrated: With the focus on animal products, hydration remains crucial. Ensure you're drinking enough water throughout the day, as some individuals may experience changes in thirst levels on this diet.

6. **Mindful Eating**: Embrace mindful eating practices. Chew your food thoroughly, savor each bite, and listen to your body's hunger and fullness cues. The cookbook might include tips on mindful eating to complement the dietary shift.

7. **Community Support:** Seek support from others who follow or have transitioned to the Carnivore Diet. Online forums, social media groups, or local communities can offer valuable advice, recipes, and moral support.

8. **Flexibility and Adaptability:** Be flexible and adapt the diet to suit your individual needs. The

cookbook's guidelines are a starting point; adjust the quantities and types of animal products based on your body's response and preferences.

CHAPTER 2

BREAKFAST DELIGHTS

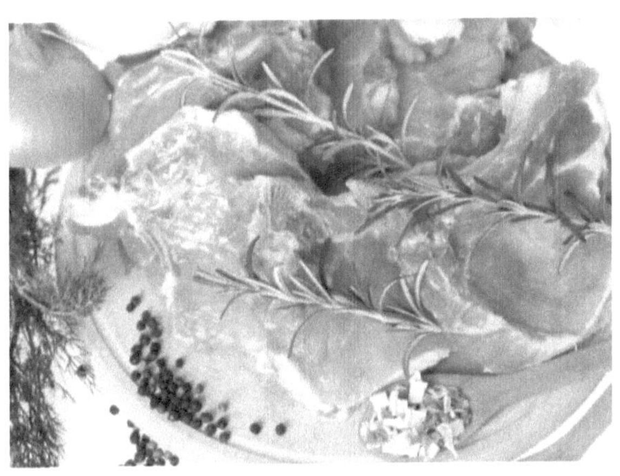

1. Carnivore Breakfast Skillet

Ingredients:

- 4 slices of bacon, chopped
- 4 large eggs
- 1/2 pound ground beef or sausage
- Salt and pepper to taste
- **Optional:** Chopped fresh herbs for garnish (parsley, chives, etc.)

Instructions:

1. Cook the diced bacon in a pan over medium heat until it becomes crispy. After taking the bacon out of the pan, put it aside. The bacon fat should stay in the skillet.
2. Add the sausage or ground beef to the pan that has the bacon fat in it. Using a spatula, break it up and heat it until it's browned and cooked through.
3. To create room for the eggs, push the cooked beef to one side of the pan.
4. Crack the eggs into the skillet's vacant area. Add a little pinch of salt and pepper to them.
5. Once the eggs are cooked to your preferred doneness, or when the whites are set but the yolks are still somewhat runny, cover the pan and continue cooking.
6. Top the pan with the crispy bacon once the eggs are cooked to your preference.
7. You may serve the breakfast skillet straight from the pan or on a dish. Garnish with chopped fresh herbs, if you'd like.

2. Salmon and Cream Cheese Roll-Ups

Ingredients:

- 4 ounces smoked salmon slices

- 4 ounces cream cheese, softened
- 2 tablespoons chopped fresh dill or chives (optional)
- Freshly ground black pepper
- Lemon wedges, for serving
- Toothpicks or cocktail sticks

Instructions:

1. Arrange the pieces of smoked salmon on a sanitized surface. To make spreading the cream cheese easier, make sure it's softened.

2. Evenly distribute a dollop of softened cream cheese over each smoked salmon piece.

3. Sprinkle fresh chives or dill over the cream cheese layer if using them. For added taste, grind some fresh black pepper and add a dash.

4. Carefully wrap each salmon slice with the cream cheese into a tight roll, starting at one end.

5. To hold each roll-up together once it has been rolled, fasten it with a cocktail stick or toothpick.

6. To slightly firm up, place the roll-ups in the refrigerator for 15 to 20 minutes.

7. Before serving, take out the toothpicks. Serve the Salmon and Cream Cheese Roll-Ups with lemon wedges on the side for a zesty garnish.

3. Bacon-Wrapped Breakfast Asparagus

Ingredients:

- 12 spears of asparagus, tough ends trimmed
- 6 slices of bacon, cut in half lengthwise
- Olive oil (for drizzling)
- Salt and pepper to taste
- Optional: Garlic powder, grated Parmesan cheese, or lemon zest for additional flavor

Instructions:

1. Set the oven temperature to 400°F, or 200°C. To make cleaning easier, line a baking sheet with parchment paper.
2. Starting from the bottom and working your way up, wrap half a piece of bacon around each spear of asparagus. Arrange the asparagus stalks with bacon on the baking sheet that has been preheated.
3. For added crispiness, drizzle a little olive oil over the wrapped asparagus. Add salt, pepper, and any other ingredients you want, such lemon zest, Parmesan cheese, or garlic powder.
4. Transfer the baking sheet to the oven, and bake for 15 to 20 minutes, or until the asparagus is soft and the bacon is crisp. To guarantee that the asparagus cooks evenly, flip it halfway through.
5. When finished, take them out of the oven and give them a minute or two to cool. Place the

Breakfast Asparagus Wrapped in Bacon onto a serving platter.

4. *Carnivore Breakfast Scramble*

Ingredients:

- Bacon or sausage
- Eggs
- Optional: Cheese (if tolerated)
- Salt and pepper to taste
- Chopped fresh herbs for garnish (optional)

Instructions:

1. In a skillet, fry the sausage or bacon until it's crispy or fully cooked.
2. Crack the eggs and scramble them with the cooked bacon or sausage in the same pan that has the rendered fat in it.
3. Add the cheese, if using, to the scramble and stir until it melts and is well blended.
4. To taste, add salt and pepper to the scramble.
5. After the scramble is cooked to your preferred consistency, move it to a platter.
6. If preferred, garnish with finely chopped fresh herbs and enjoy this meal full of protein!

5. *Carnivore Breakfast Burrito*

Ingredients:

- Large lettuce leaves or cabbage leaves (for wrapping)
- 4 large eggs
- 4 slices of bacon or sausage
- Sliced deli meat (turkey, ham, roast beef, etc.)
- Optional: Cheese (if tolerated)
- Salt and pepper to taste
- Hot sauce or spices (optional)

Instructions:

1. Over medium heat, scramble the eggs in a pan until the appropriate consistency is achieved. Add salt and pepper for seasoning.
2. In another pan, fry the sausage or bacon until it's crispy or fully cooked.
3. Spread out the big cabbage or lettuce leaves evenly. These will function as the burrito's "tortilla".
4. Arrange the sliced deli meat, cooked eggs, and bacon or sausage among the lettuce or cabbage leaves. Place cheese on top if using it.
5. If you want more taste, add your favorite spices or spicy sauce.
6. To create a burrito, gently fold the edges of the lettuce or cabbage leaves over the contents.

7. Savor the Carnivore Breakfast Burrito immediately.

6. Carnivore Breakfast Frittata

Ingredients:

- 8 large eggs
- 1/2 pound ground breakfast sausage or diced bacon
- 1/2 cup shredded cheese (if tolerated, optional)
- Salt and pepper to taste
- Olive oil or bacon fat for cooking

Instructions:

1. Set the oven temperature to 175°C, or 350°F.
2. Cook the breakfast sausage or chopped bacon in an oven-safe pan over medium heat until it is browned and well cooked. If desirable, remove extra fat; if not, leave it in the pan for flavor.
3. Thoroughly whisk the eggs in a mixing basin until well blended. Add salt and pepper to taste while preparing the eggs.
4. Evenly distribute the cooked meat across the skillet. Sprinkle cheese on top of the meat if using it.

5. Pour the meat and cheese mixture in the pan with the whisked eggs. To uniformly spread the ingredients, whisk gently.

6. Allow the mixture to cook over medium heat for three to four minutes, or until the edges begin to firm slightly.

7. Place the pan in the oven that has been prepared, and bake for 12 to 15 minutes, or until the frittata is cooked through and it is golden on top.

8. After the frittata is done, take it out of the oven and allow it to cool for a little while. After slicing it into wedges, serve.

7. *Steak and Cheese Omelet*

Ingredients:

- 2 large eggs
- 4 ounces cooked steak, thinly sliced
- 1/4 cup shredded cheese (such as cheddar or mozzarella)
- Salt and pepper to taste
- Butter or oil for cooking

Instructions:

1. If the steak hasn't been cooked yet, cook it to your desired doneness (grill, pan-sear, etc.) and cut it into thin slices.

2. Beat the eggs well with a whisk in a bowl. To taste, add salt and pepper for seasoning.

3. Add butter or oil to a nonstick skillet that is heated to medium heat. Pour the beaten eggs into the skillet after it's hot.

4. Evenly spread the thinly sliced steak and shredded cheese over one side of the omelet as the edges begin to firm.

5. Gently fold the remaining omelet over the filling of cheese and meat using a spatula. Cook for a minute more, or until the omelet is well cooked and the cheese has melted.

6. Transfer the cheese and steak omelet to a platter and start serving right away.

8. Scrumptious Carnivore Omelets

Classic Bacon and Cheese Omelet

Ingredients:

- 2 large eggs
- 2 slices of bacon, cooked and crumbled
- 1/4 cup shredded cheese (cheddar, mozzarella, etc.)
- Salt and pepper to taste
- Butter or oil for cooking

Instructions:

1. In a bowl, whisk together the eggs and season with salt and pepper.
2. Melt butter or oil in a nonstick pan over medium heat.
3. Transfer the whisked eggs into the skillet and let them begin firming up.
4. Top half of the omelet with shredded cheese and crumbled bacon.
5. Fold the remaining omelet over the filling, then continue cooking it until the cheese has melted.
6. Serve the heated Bacon and Cheese Omelet.

Sausage and Mushroom Omelet

Ingredients:

- 2 large eggs
- 2 cooked sausage links, sliced
- 1/4 cup sliced mushrooms
- Salt and pepper to taste
- Butter or oil for cooking

Instructions:

1. In a bowl, whisk together the eggs and season with salt and pepper.
2. Melt butter or oil in a nonstick pan over medium heat.

3. Transfer the whisked eggs into the skillet and let them begin firming up.

4. Top one half of the omelet with the sausage slices and the mushrooms.

5. After folding the second half over the filling, fry the omelet until it is well cooked.

6. Serve the heated Omelet with sausage and mushrooms.

Steak and Spinach Omelet

Ingredients:

- 2 large eggs
- 2-3 ounces cooked steak, diced
- Handful of fresh spinach leaves
- Salt and pepper to taste
- Butter or oil for cooking

Instructions:

1. In a bowl, whisk together the eggs and season with salt and pepper.

2. Melt butter or oil in a nonstick pan over medium heat.

3. Transfer the whisked eggs into the skillet and let them begin firming up.

4. Top one half of the omelet with the cubed steak and fresh spinach leaves.

5. Once the omelet is ready, fold the remaining half over the filling.

6. Serve the hot spinach and steak omelet.

9. Homemade Carnivore Breakfast Sausages

Ingredients:

- 1 pound ground pork or beef
- 1 teaspoon salt
- 1/2 teaspoon black pepper
- 1/2 teaspoon ground sage
- 1/4 teaspoon garlic powder
- 1/4 teaspoon onion powder
- Pinch of cayenne pepper (optional, for heat)
- Cooking fat for frying (such as bacon fat or butter)

Instructions:

1. Place the ground beef or pork, onion powder, garlic powder, sage, salt, and pepper in a mixing bowl. Add cayenne pepper, if desired. Once the spices are uniformly incorporated into the meat, carefully mix.

2. Form the spiced beef mixture into patties by dividing it into pieces. Depending on your desire, you may either flatten them into patties or shape them into classic sausage forms.

3. Add a tablespoon of cooking fat to a pan that is heated to medium heat. The sausage patties should be added to the heating skillet. Cook for approximately 4–5 minutes on each side, or until the outsides are beautifully browned and the internal temperature reaches 160°F (71°C).
4. After the handmade Carnivore Breakfast Sausages are cooked through, place them on a serving platter and savor them warm.

10. Creamy Steak and Eggs

Ingredients:

- 8 ounces steak (sirloin, ribeye, or your preferred cut)
- 4 large eggs
- 2 tablespoons butter
- Salt and pepper to taste
- Optional: Heavy cream or cream cheese for added creaminess

Instructions:

1. Season both sides of the steak with salt and pepper.
2. Turn the heat up to medium-high in a skillet. Spoon in one tablespoon of butter into the pan. When it's heated, add the steak and cook it to the

doneness you prefer. Before slicing the steak thinly across the grain, take it out of the pan and let it rest for a few minutes.

3. Add one more tablespoon of butter to the same skillet. Once the eggs are cracked into the pan, cook them as you would like: fried, scrambled, or sunny-side up.

4. Arrange the cooked eggs next to the cut steak on a platter. If preferred, top the steak with a dollop of heavy cream or cream cheese for extra smoothness.

5. Serve the steak and eggs right away after adding more salt and pepper, if necessary.

CHAPTER 3

1. Carnivor Beef Lettuce Wraps

Ingredients:

- 1 pound ground beef (preferably grass-fed)
- 2 cloves garlic, minced
- Salt and pepper to taste
- Iceberg lettuce leaves (or any large lettuce leaves suitable for wrapping)
- Optional toppings: Chopped green onions, sliced radishes, or hot sauce

Instructions:

1. Cook the ground beef in a pan over medium-high heat, breaking it up with a spatula as it cooks. When the meat is browned and well cooked, add the minced garlic to the pan and cook it further. Remove any extra fat if preferred.
2. To taste, add salt and pepper to the cooked meat. To fully incorporate the seasoning, mix well.

3. Rinse the lettuce leaves and pat dry. Form the meat mixture into "wraps" using the bigger, more robust leaves.

4. Place a little amount of the spiced ground beef onto every leaf of lettuce.

5. You may top the beef with sliced radishes, chopped green onions, or even a sprinkle of spicy sauce, if you'd like.

6. To make lettuce wraps, roll or fold the leaves around the meat. If necessary, fasten them with toothpicks and proceed to serve immediately.

2. Grilled Chicken Thighs with Lemon-Herb Butter

Ingredients:

- 4 chicken thighs, bone-in and skin-on
- 2 tablespoons olive oil
- Salt and pepper to taste

For Lemon-Herb Butter:

- 4 tablespoons unsalted butter, softened
- 2 tablespoons chopped fresh herbs (such as parsley, thyme, or rosemary)
- Zest of 1 lemon
- Salt and pepper to taste

Instructions:

1. Turn the heat up to medium-high on your grill.
2. Use paper towels to pat dry the chicken thighs. Lightly coat them in olive oil and liberally sprinkle with salt and pepper.
3. Combine melted butter, lemon zest, chopped fresh herbs, salt, and pepper in a bowl. Stir until well mixed. Put away.
4. Skin-side down, put the chicken thighs on the prepared grill. Grill until the internal temperature reaches 165°F (74°C) and the skin is crispy and golden, approximately 5 to 6 minutes on each side.
5. After the chicken thighs are thoroughly cooked, place them on a platter. While the chicken thighs are still hot, place a dollop of the prepared Lemon-Herb Butter on top of each one, letting the butter to melt slightly.
6. Before serving, let the chicken thighs rest for a few minutes. As a result, the tastes might combine. Serve the Lemon-Herb Butter Grilled Chicken Thighs hot.

3. Savory Beef Bone Broth Soup

Ingredients:

- Beef bones (preferably marrow bones or soup bones)

- Water
- Salt (optional)
- Pepper (optional)
- Optional add-ins: Fresh herbs, garlic cloves, onions, celery, or carrots (for flavor, but avoid if following strict carnivore guidelines)

Instructions:

Set the oven temperature to 400°F, or 200°C. The beef bones should be roasted in the oven for 30 to 40 minutes, or until they are golden brown, after placing them on a baking sheet. This process improves the broth's taste.

2. After the bones are cooked, put them in a big saucepan and add water to cover. After bringing the water to a boil, lower the heat to a low simmer. If any foam comes to the top, skim it off.

3. Taste and add salt and pepper, if required. For extra taste, you may also add any optional herbs or veggies; but, if you're strictly adhering to the carnivorous diet, leave them out.

4. Simmer the broth on low heat for four to six hours, or, if time permits, for up to twenty-four hours. The tastes and minerals are extracted from the bones by this lengthy boiling.

5. To get rid of the bones and other particles, drain the broth into a clean container using cheesecloth or a fine-mesh strainer after it has simmered.

6. Spoon the flavorful Beef Bone Broth Soup into a dish for a filling and healthy meal.

4. Seared Pork Tenderloin with Dijon Mustard

Ingredients:

- 1 pork tenderloin
- Salt and pepper to taste
- 2 tablespoons Dijon mustard
- 1 tablespoon olive oil
- Optional: Fresh herbs (rosemary, thyme) for garnish

Instructions:

1. Using paper towels, pat dry the pork tenderloin and liberally season it on both sides.
2. Using a brush or spoon, evenly cover the whole surface of the pork tenderloin with the Dijon mustard.
3. Turn up the heat to medium-high in a skillet or frying pan. Fill the pan with olive oil and let it warm up.
4. Add the pork tenderloin to the skillet when it has heated up. Cook it for about 3–4 minutes on each side, or until a golden-brown crust forms.
5. Depending on your choice, use a meat thermometer to make sure the pork achieves an

internal temperature of 160°F (71°C) for medium-rare or 145°F (63°C) for medium-rare. Take it off the heat and give it some time to rest.
6. Slice the seared pork tenderloin and place it on a serving tray when it has rested. If preferred, garnish with fresh herbs and serve.

5. Bacon-Wrapped Shrimp Skewers

Ingredients:

- 12 large shrimp, peeled and deveined
- 6 slices of bacon, cut in half
- Wooden or metal skewers
- Salt and pepper to taste
- Optional: Garlic powder, smoked paprika, or chili powder for extra flavor

Instructions:

1. Use paper towels to pat dry the shrimp, then sprinkle them with a little amount of salt and pepper. For added taste, feel free to add more spices like chili powder, smoky paprika, or garlic powder.
2. Take a half-slice of bacon and wrap it around each shrimp. To ensure the bacon remains in place, thread the shrimp that have been wrapped in bacon onto the skewers.

3. Turn the heat up to medium-high on your grill or prepare a grill pan over the stove.

4. Transfer the shrimp skewers wrapped in bacon to the grill or grill pan. Grill until the bacon is crispy and the shrimp are pink and opaque, approximately 2 to 3 minutes each side, flipping them over regularly.

5. Take the Shrimp Skewers wrapped in bacon off the grill or pan after they are cooked through. Before serving, allow them to cool for a minute or two.

6. Herb-Crusted Lamb Chops

Ingredients:

- 4 lamb chops (loin or rib chops), about 1 inch thick
- 2 tablespoons olive oil
- Salt and pepper to taste

For the Herb Crust:

- 2 tablespoons fresh rosemary leaves, finely chopped
- 2 tablespoons fresh thyme leaves, finely chopped
- 2 cloves garlic, minced
- Zest of 1 lemon
- 2 tablespoons olive oil

- Salt and pepper to taste

Instructions:

1. Set the oven temperature to 400°F, or 200°C.
2. Add the olive oil, minced garlic, chopped rosemary, thyme, and lemon zest to a bowl. Well combined to create a paste. To taste, add more salt and pepper to the mixture.
3. Use paper towels to pat dry the lamb chops. Sprinkle salt and pepper on both lamb chop sides.
4. Add two teaspoons of olive oil to an ovenproof skillet and heat it over medium-high heat. When the lamb chops are heated, sear them for two to three minutes on each side, or until a golden-brown crust forms.
5. Turn off the heat source for the skillet. Evenly coat the upper surface of every lamb chop with the herb crust mixture.
6. Put the lamb chops and skillet into the oven that has been prepared. For medium-rare, bake for 8 to 10 minutes; vary cooking time according to desired doneness.
7. After the lamb chops are cooked to your liking, take them out of the oven and give them a few minutes to rest before serving.

Contd

7. Sliced Roast Turkey with Avocado Salsa

Ingredients:

- 1 pound roast turkey, thinly sliced
- 2 ripe avocados, diced
- 1 tomato, diced
- 1/4 red onion, finely chopped
- 1 jalapeño pepper, seeded and finely chopped (optional)
- Juice of 1 lime
- 2 tablespoons chopped fresh cilantro
- Salt and pepper to taste

Instructions:

1. Diced avocados, diced tomato, finely chopped red onion, jalapeño pepper (if used), lime juice, chopped cilantro, and salt and pepper should all be combined in a mixing bowl. Toss the ingredients gently to ensure uniform mixing.

2. Transfer the roast turkey slices, thinly cut, to a serving tray.

3. Drizzle the sliced roast turkey with a large amount of the prepared avocado salsa.

4. For added taste, you may add more fresh cilantro or lime wedges as a garnish to the meal.

8. Grilled Chicken Salad with Bacon

Ingredients:

- 2 boneless, skinless chicken breasts
- Salt and pepper to taste
- 4-6 slices of bacon
- Mixed salad greens (lettuce, spinach, arugula, etc.)
- Cherry tomatoes, halved
- Cucumber, sliced
- Red onion, thinly sliced (optional)

Dressing Ingredients:

- 3 tablespoons olive oil
- 2 tablespoons apple cider vinegar
- 1 tablespoon Dijon mustard
- 1 clove garlic, minced
- Salt and pepper to taste

Instructions:

1. Use salt and pepper to season the chicken breasts. Grill the chicken for approximately 6-7 minutes on each side, or until it is cooked through, on a prepared grill or grill pan over medium-high heat. After grilling, let the chicken rest for a few minutes before slicing it into strips.

2. Cook the bacon in a pan over medium heat until it crisps up. After taking the bacon out of the pan, drain any excess oil by placing it on a dish covered

with paper towels. Crumble the bacon into tiny bits when it has cooled.

3. Combine the cucumber slices, cherry tomatoes, thinly sliced red onion (if using), and mixed salad greens in a big bowl. Gently toss the salad to combine the ingredients.

4. To create the dressing, combine the olive oil, Dijon mustard, apple cider vinegar, chopped garlic, salt, and pepper in a small bowl.

5. Top the mixed salad with the grilled chicken pieces and crumbled bacon. Serve the dressing on the side or drizzle it over the salad.

9. Beef and Vegetable Skewers

Ingredients:

- 1 pound beef steak (such as sirloin or ribeye), cut into cubes
- Assorted vegetables (bell peppers, onions, zucchini, cherry tomatoes, mushrooms, etc.), cut into chunks
- Wooden or metal skewers (if using wooden skewers, soak them in water for 30 minutes before assembling to prevent burning)
- Olive oil
- Salt and pepper to taste
- **Optional:** Garlic powder, smoked paprika, or herbs for extra flavor

Instructions:

1. Roughly chop the beef steak into equal-sized pieces. Chop the mixed veggies into pieces that are appropriate for skewering.

2. Alternate between the steak and the veggies as you thread the beef cubes and other vegetables onto the skewers. To ensure consistent cooking, leave some space between each piece.

3. To enhance flavor, brush the skewers with olive oil and season them with salt, pepper, and any other herbs or spices you want.

4. Turn the heat up to medium-high on your grill or prepare a grill pan over the stove.

5. Set up the grill pan or grill skewers. Grill the meat for 3–4 minutes on each side, turning it from time to time, or until the steak is cooked to your desired doneness and the veggies are soft and gently browned.

6. Take the beef and vegetable skewers from the grill once they are done. Before serving, let them have a minute or two to rest.

10. Grilled Lemon Garlic Salmon

Ingredients:

- 2 salmon filets

- 2 tablespoons olive oil
- 2 cloves garlic, minced
- Zest and juice of 1 lemon
- Salt and pepper to taste
- Fresh parsley (optional, for garnish)

Instructions:

1. Turn the heat up to medium-high on your grill.
2. Combine the lemon zest, lemon juice, olive oil, chopped garlic, salt, and pepper in a bowl.
3. Lay the salmon filets in a shallow plate after petting them dry. Make sure the salmon is covered on all sides by pouring the marinade over it. Give it a good 15 to 20 minutes to marinade.
4. To keep the grill grates from sticking, lightly oil them. With the skin side down, place the salmon filets on the grill. Cook under the grill for 4–5 minutes on each side, or until the food is tender and flakes readily with a fork.
5. Take the salmon off the grill when it's done. If preferred, garnish with fresh parsley and serve immediately.

CHAPTER 4

SATISFYING DINNER RECIPES

1. Ribeye Steak with Blue Cheese Butter

Ingredients:

- 2 Ribeye steaks (about 1 inch thick)
- Salt and pepper to taste
- Olive oil (for grilling)
- 4 tablespoons unsalted butter, softened
- 2-3 tablespoons crumbled blue cheese
- Fresh parsley, finely chopped (optional, for garnish)

Instructions:

1. Place the crumbled blue cheese and melted butter in a small bowl. Mix thoroughly, stirring. The quantity of blue cheese may be changed to suit your taste in terms of flavor strength. Put away.

2. Turn up the heat to high on your grill or grill pan.

3. Use paper towels to pat dry the ribeye steaks. Give the steaks a liberal amount of salt and pepper on both sides.

4. To keep the steaks from sticking, lightly coat them with olive oil on both sides. The steaks should be placed on the heated grill or grill pan. For medium-rare, grill for around 4–5 minutes on each side, altering the cooking time according to your preferred degree of doneness.

5. Take the steaks from the grill and let them rest for a few minutes when they are cooked to your preference. While the steaks are still hot, place a large dollop of the made Blue Cheese Butter on top of each one, letting it melt slightly.

6. If preferred, top the steaks with finely chopped fresh parsley for extra taste and a flash of color. Serve the Blue Cheese Butter Ribeye Steaks immediately.

2. Baked Chicken Thighs with Garlic and Herbs

Ingredients:

- 4 bone-in, skin-on chicken thighs
- 4 cloves garlic, minced
- 2 tablespoons olive oil
- 1 teaspoon dried thyme
- 1 teaspoon dried rosemary

- Salt and pepper to taste
- Fresh parsley for garnish (optional)

Instructions:

1. Set the oven temperature to 400°F, or 200°C.
2. Use paper towels to pat dry the chicken thighs. On both sides, liberally season them with salt and pepper.
3. Combine the minced garlic, olive oil, dried rosemary, and dried thyme in a small bowl.
4. Transfer the chicken thighs to a baking dish or a parchment paper-lined baking sheet. Apply a uniform layer of the garlic and herb mixture to each chicken thigh.
5. Slide the chicken thighs-filled baking dish into the oven that has been prepared. Bake the chicken thighs for 30 to 35 minutes, or until the skin is crispy and golden brown and the meat is cooked through.
6. Make sure the chicken achieves an internal temperature of at least 165°F (74°C) by using a meat thermometer.
7. Take the chicken thighs out of the oven once they've roasted. If preferred, garnish with fresh parsley and serve hot.

3. Seared Salmon with Lemon-Dill Sauce

Ingredients:

- 2 salmon filets
- Salt and pepper to taste
- 2 tablespoons olive oil

For the Lemon-Dill Sauce:

- 1/4 cup mayonnaise
- 1 tablespoon fresh dill, chopped
- Zest and juice of 1 lemon
- 1 clove garlic, minced
- Salt and pepper to taste

Instructions:

1. Using paper towels, pat dry the salmon filets. Sprinkle salt and pepper on the filets' two sides.
2. Add olive oil to a pan and heat it to medium-high heat.
3. Place the salmon filets, skin-side down, in the skillet when it has heated up. Sear the skin side for 4–5 minutes, or until crispy. Once the filets are cooked through, flip them over and cook for a further two to three minutes on the other side. Depending on the thickness of the filets, adjust the cooking time.
4. Make the sauce while the fish cooks. Combine the mayonnaise, lemon zest, lemon juice, minced

garlic, chopped fresh dill, salt, and pepper in a small bowl.

5. Take the salmon out of the pan when it's done. Spoon the Lemon-Dill Sauce over the salmon filets or serve it as a side dish for dipping.

4. Spice-Rubbed Pork Ribs

Ingredients:

- 2 racks of pork ribs
- 2 tablespoons brown sugar (optional, omit for strict carnivore)
- 2 tablespoons paprika
- 1 tablespoon garlic powder
- 1 tablespoon onion powder
- 1 tablespoon ground cumin
- 1 tablespoon chili powder
- 1 tablespoon black pepper
- 1 tablespoon salt
- 2 tablespoons olive oil or preferred cooking fat

Instructions:

1. If required, take off the membrane below the ribs. Using paper towels, pat the ribs dry.
2. To make the spice rub, combine the paprika, black pepper, cumin, chili powder, garlic powder,

onion powder, brown sugar (if using), and salt in a bowl.

3. Use olive oil or your favorite cooking fat to coat the ribs on both sides. Sprinkle the ribs with a liberal amount of the spice rub, rubbing the spices into the meat to make sure they stick.

4. Refrigerate the seasoned ribs for at least two to four hours, or better yet, overnight, to enhance their taste. Wrap them in plastic wrap.

5. Set the temperature of your oven to 300°F (150°C) or turn on your grill to indirect heat.

6. If using a grill, put the ribs on it and cook it indirectly. The ribs should be tender and the internal temperature should reach between 145 and 160°F (63 and 71°C) after two to three hours of grilling, with periodic flipping. Place the ribs on a foil-lined baking sheet and bake for the same length of time if you're using an oven.

7. Before slicing and serving, let the ribs rest for a few minutes after they are cooked through and tender.

5. Grilled Shrimp Scampi

Ingredients:

- 1 pound large shrimp, peeled and deveined
- 4 tablespoons butter, melted
- 4 cloves garlic, minced

- Zest and juice of 1 lemon
- 2 tablespoons fresh parsley, chopped
- Salt and pepper to taste
- Olive oil (for grilling)
- Optional: Red pepper flakes for a spicy kick

Instructions:

1. Use paper towels to gently pat dry the shrimp. If using wooden skewers, soak them in water for half an hour before using. Thread the shrimp onto the skewers, being sure to pierce through both the head and the tail of each shrimp.
2. To make the marinade, add the chopped parsley, lemon zest, lemon juice, minced garlic, melted butter, salt, pepper, and red pepper flakes (if using) to a bowl and mix thoroughly.
3. Put the shrimp skewers that have been strung onto a shallow tray or plate. Coat the shrimp equally by brushing them with the garlic butter mixture. Give them ten to fifteen minutes to marinade.
4. Turn the heat up to medium-high on your grill.
5. To keep the grill grates from sticking, give them a little olive oil brushing. Put the skewers of shrimp onto the grill. The shrimp should be pink and fully cooked after grilling them for two to three minutes on each side, rotating once.

6. Take the shrimp skewers from the grill once they are done. If preferred, top the hot Grilled Shrimp Scampi with extra lemon wedges for squeezing.

6. Herb-Marinated Lamb Kebabs

Ingredients:

- 1 ½ pounds lamb leg or shoulder, cut into cubes
- Wooden or metal skewers (if using wooden skewers, soak them in water for 30 minutes before using)

For the Marinade:

- 3 cloves garlic, minced
- 2 tablespoons olive oil
- 2 tablespoons fresh rosemary, chopped
- 2 tablespoons fresh thyme, chopped
- Zest and juice of 1 lemon
- Salt and pepper to taste

Instructions:

1. Combine the minced garlic, olive oil, lemon zest, lemon juice, chopped thyme, and rosemary in a bowl. Season with salt and pepper. To make the marinade, thoroughly mix.

2. Transfer the cubed lamb to a tray or shallow dish. Make sure the lamb is uniformly covered by pouring the marinade over it. To let the flavors to infuse, cover the dish with plastic wrap and refrigerate for at least 2-4 hours, or preferably overnight.

3. Turn the heat up to medium-high on your grill.

4. To ensure consistent cooking, thread the marinated lamb cubes onto the skewers, leaving a little gap between each piece.

5. To keep the grill grates from sticking, lightly oil them. Chargrill the lamb skewers over the heat. Cook, rotating regularly, for 3–4 minutes on each side, or until the lamb is cooked to your preferred doneness.

6. Take the lamb kebabs from the grill after they are well cooked. Before serving, let them rest for a few minutes.

7. Braised Beef Short Ribs

Ingredients:

- 4 pounds beef short ribs, bone-in
- Salt and pepper to taste
- 2 tablespoons olive oil
- 1 onion, diced
- 2 carrots, diced
- 3 cloves garlic, minced

- 2 cups beef broth
- 1 cup red wine (optional, can replace with beef broth)
- 2 sprigs fresh thyme
- 2 sprigs fresh rosemary
- 2 bay leaves

Instructions:

1. Set the oven's temperature to 325°F (163°C).
2. Use paper towels to pat dry the beef short ribs. On both sides, liberally season them with salt and pepper.
3. Turn the heat up to medium-high in a Dutch oven or ovenproof pot. Grease the saucepan with olive oil. Short ribs should be seared in batches so that they have a rich golden-brown crust all over. After removing the ribs, put them aside.
4. Add the minced garlic, carrots, and chopped onion to the same saucepan. Let them cook for a few minutes until they start to become tender.
5. Add the red wine (if using) and beef broth, scraping off any browned pieces from the pot's bottom.
6. Put back into the saucepan the short ribs that have seared. Add bay leaves, sprigs of rosemary, and fresh thyme. Simmer the liquid for a while.
7. Place a cover on the saucepan and place it in the oven that has been prepared. The short ribs should

be braised for three to four hours, or until the meat is falling off the bone tender.

8. Take the short ribs out of the oven when they're done. Spoon the fragrant sauce and veggies over the top of the hot Braised Beef Short Ribs.

8. Juicy Ribeye Steak with Garlic Butter

Ingredients:

- 2 Ribeye steaks (about 1 inch thick)
- Salt and pepper to taste
- 2 tablespoons olive oil
- 4 tablespoons unsalted butter, softened
- 4 cloves garlic, minced
- 2 tablespoons fresh parsley, chopped
- **Optional:** Red pepper flakes for a hint of spice

Instructions:

1. Using paper towels, pat dry the ribeye steaks. Add a liberal amount of salt and pepper on both sides.

2. Turn up the heat to medium-high in a skillet or grill pan. Set the grill to high heat if you want to use one.

3. Drizzle the grill grates or skillet with olive oil. Add the ribeye steaks when they're heated. For medium-rare, cook for approximately 4–5 minutes

on each side, modifying the cooking time according to your desired degree of doneness.

4. Combine the softened butter, minced garlic, parsley, and red pepper flakes (if using) in a small bowl. To make the garlic butter, thoroughly mix.

5. After the steaks are done to your satisfaction, take them off the grill or pan and allow them to rest for a few minutes on a plate or cutting board.

6. Top each steak with a dollop of the garlic butter while it is still resting. Let it soften a little over the sizzling steaks.

7. Drizzle the Garlic Butter and any collected juices over the juicy ribeye steaks on the plate. For freshness, you may optionally add additional chopped parsley as a garnish.

9. Baked Salmon with Lemon and Dill

Ingredients:

- 2 salmon filets
- Salt and pepper to taste
- 2 tablespoons olive oil
- Zest of 1 lemon
- Juice of 1 lemon
- 2 tablespoons fresh dill, chopped
- **Optional:** Slices of lemon for garnish

Instructions:

1. Set the oven temperature to 375°F, or 190°C.

2. Use paper towels to pat dry the salmon filets. Sprinkle salt and pepper on the filets' two sides.

3. Combine the olive oil, lemon juice, zest, and chopped fresh dill in a small bowl. To make the lemon and dill combination, thoroughly combine.

4. Arrange the salmon filets on a parchment paper-lined baking sheet. Toss each filet in the lemon and dill mixture, covering well.

5. Put the salmon-containing baking sheet in the oven that has been preheated. Depending on the thickness of the filets, bake for 12 to 15 minutes, or until the salmon is cooked through and flake easily with a fork.

6. Take the salmon out of the oven after it has roasted. For appearance purposes, you may choose to add more fresh dill or lemon slices to the baked salmon with dill.

10. Pork Chops with Mushroom Gravy

Ingredients:

- 4 pork chops (bone-in or boneless)
- Salt and pepper to taste
- 2 tablespoons olive oil or cooking fat
- 1 onion, finely chopped
- 8 oz mushrooms, sliced

- 2 cloves garlic, minced
- 1 cup beef or chicken broth
- 1/2 cup heavy cream or coconut cream (for dairy-free option)
- 1 tablespoon fresh thyme leaves (or 1 teaspoon dried thyme)
- 1 tablespoon butter (optional, omit for dairy-free or use ghee)
- 2 tablespoons chopped fresh parsley for garnish

Instructions:

1. Using paper towels, pat dry the pork chops. Add salt and pepper to the pork chops' two sides.

2. In a skillet over medium-high heat, warm up some olive oil or cooking fat. When the skillet is heated, add the pork chops. Sear till golden brown, approximately 3–4 minutes each side. The pork chops should be taken out of the griddle and placed aside.

3. If necessary, add a little more oil to the same skillet. Sauté the chopped onion until it becomes transparent. Add the minced garlic and cut mushrooms. Sauté the mushrooms until they are soft and beginning to become golden.

4. Add the beef or chicken stock, being sure to scrape down the skillet's bottom to achieve a deglaze. Add the fresh leaves of thyme. Simmer the mixture for a while.

5. Turn down the heat to low and mix in the coconut or heavy cream. To slightly thicken the sauce, let it boil gently for a few minutes.

6. Add the cooked pork chops and any collected juices back to the skillet. Simmer the pork chops in the mushroom gravy for a further five to seven minutes, or until they are well cooked.

7. If desired, add a tablespoon of butter and swirl it in to give it more richness. Before serving, top the pork chops with mushroom gravy with finely chopped fresh parsley.

CHAPTER 5

SNACKS AND APPETIZERS

1. Bacon-Wrapped Jalapeño Poppers

Ingredients:

- 12 fresh jalapeño peppers
- 8 oz cream cheese, softened
- 1 cup shredded cheddar cheese
- 12 slices bacon, cut in half
- Toothpicks (optional)

Instructions:

1. Turn the oven on to 375°F, or 190°C. After cleaning, cut the jalapeño peppers in half lengthwise. The seeds and membranes may be removed using a spoon or knife. If you are sensitive to heat, wear gloves while handling the spicy seeds.

2. Gently stir the melted cream cheese and the shredded cheddar cheese together in a bowl until well mixed.

3. Evenly spoon the cheese mixture into each side of the jalapeños to fill them up.

4. Using a half-slice of bacon, enclose each filled jalapeño half, being sure to secure it around the pepper. If necessary, you may fasten the bacon with toothpicks.

5. Arrange the jalapeño poppers wrapped in bacon on a baking sheet covered with parchment paper. Bake for 20 to 25 minutes, or until the peppers are soft and the bacon is crispy, in a preheated oven.

6. Take the jalapeño poppers out of the oven once they've roasted. Before serving, let them cool for a few minutes.

2. Sliced Roast Beef Roll-Ups

Ingredients:

- Thinly sliced roast beef (deli-sliced or homemade)
- Cream cheese, softened
- Pickles, sliced into thin strips
- Mustard (optional)
- Toothpicks (optional, for securing roll-ups)

Instructions:

1. Arrange the roast beef slices thinly on a sanitized surface.

2. Cover each roast beef slice with a thin coating of softened cream cheese.

3. Top each roast beef slice with a strip of sliced pickle on one end.

4. You may spread a tiny coating of mustard directly on the pickle strip or over the cream cheese, if you'd like.

5. Tightly coil up each roast beef slice, beginning with the pickle strip at the end.

6. Use toothpicks to hold the roll-ups in place if necessary to prevent them from unwrapping.

7. Place the cut roast beef roll-ups onto a platter and start serving right away.

3. Creamy Chicken Liver Pâté

Ingredients:

- 1 pound chicken livers, cleaned and trimmed
- 1/2 cup unsalted butter
- 1 onion, finely chopped
- 2 cloves garlic, minced
- 1/4 cup brandy or dry sherry
- 1/4 teaspoon ground thyme
- 1/4 teaspoon ground nutmeg
- Salt and pepper to taste

- **Optional**: Fresh herbs (parsley or thyme) for garnish

Instructions:

1. Use paper towels to gently dry the chicken livers after rinsing them in cold water. If there are any green areas or connective tissues, remove them.
2. Melt two tablespoons of butter in a pan over medium heat. Add the minced garlic and chopped onions. The onions should be transparent and aromatic after sautéing.
3. Push the garlic and onions over to one side of the pan. When the chicken livers are browned on the surface but still somewhat pink inside, add them to the skillet and cook for 3 to 4 minutes on each side. Make cautious not to overcook them so they stay soft.
4. To deglaze the pan and remove any browned pieces, pour in the brandy or dry sherry and scrape the bottom. To let the alcohol evaporate, cook for one more minute.
5. Place the cooked chicken livers in a food processor together with the onions and garlic. Add the ground nutmeg, ground thyme, ground pepper, and salt. Blend till creamy and smooth.
6. After tasting the pâté, adjust the seasoning to your taste, adding more salt, pepper, or spices if necessary.

7. Spoon the Creamy Chicken Liver Pâté into individual ramekins or a serving plate. Garnish with fresh herbs, if desired. Before serving, cover and chill for a minimum of two hours to enable the flavors to mingle.

8. As a tasty appetizer or snack, serve the chilled pâté with cucumber slices or low-carb crackers.

4. Spicy Buffalo Chicken Wings

Ingredients:

- 2 lbs chicken wings, split at joints, tips removed
- Salt and pepper to taste
- 1/2 cup hot sauce (such as Frank's RedHot or your preferred brand)
- 1/4 cup unsalted butter, melted
- 1 tablespoon vinegar (white or apple cider)
- Optional: Blue cheese dressing or ranch dressing for serving
- **Optional**: Celery sticks for serving

Instructions:

Set the oven temperature to 400°F, or 200°C. Use parchment paper to line a baking sheet.

2. Use paper towels to gently pat dry the chicken wings. To taste, add salt and pepper to season them.

3. Arrange the spiced chicken wings in a single layer on the baking sheet that has been ready. Bake for 45 to 50 minutes in a preheated oven, rotating them halfway through, or until crispy and golden brown.

4. Combine the vinegar, melted butter, and spicy sauce in a mixing bowl. Mix until everything is fully blended.

5. After the chicken wings are baked, move them to a sanitized basin. After adding the buffalo sauce to the wings, toss them around to cover them completely.

6. Present the hot Buffalo Chicken Wings on a plate and go straight ahead and serve them with ranch or blue cheese dressing for dipping. Serve with celery sticks on the side, if desired.

5. Cheese-Stuffed Mini Bell Peppers

Ingredients:

- 12 mini bell peppers (assorted colors if available)
- 8 oz cream cheese, softened
- 1 cup shredded cheddar cheese
- 1/4 cup grated Parmesan cheese
- 2 green onions, finely chopped
- 1 teaspoon garlic powder
- Salt and pepper to taste

- **Optional:** Smoked paprika or fresh herbs for garnish

Instructions:

1. Turn the oven on to 375°F, or 190°C. Slice off the tops of the tiny bell peppers, removing the membranes and seeds.
2. Place the melted cream cheese, grated Parmesan cheese, shredded cheddar cheese, finely chopped green onions, garlic powder, salt, and pepper in a mixing bowl. Stir until well mixed.
3. Spoon or pipette the cheese mixture into each small bell pepper, carefully pressing it in to fill the peppers.
4. Transfer the filled small bell peppers to a parchment paper-lined baking sheet. Bake for 15 to 20 minutes in a preheated oven, or until the cheese is melted and faintly browned on top and the peppers are soft.
5. Take the Cheese-Stuffed Mini Bell Peppers out of the oven once they have roasted. As an optional garnish, top them with fresh herbs or smoked paprika. Serve the peppers heated as a tasty snack or appetizer.

6. Smoked Sausage Bites with Mustard

Ingredients:

- 1 pound smoked sausage (such as kielbasa or any preferred variety)
- Dijon mustard or whole-grain mustard for dipping

Instructions:

1. Cut the smoked sausage into 1/2-inch-thick rounds or diagonal slices that are bite-sized.
2. Turn up the heat to medium-high in a skillet or grill pan. When the pan is heated, add the sliced smoked sausage.
3. Cook the bite-sized pieces of smoked sausage for three to four minutes on each side, or until they are well browned and thoroughly cooked.
4. Spoon the cooked Smoked Sausage Bites onto a tray or serving dish. Warm them up and serve with whole-grain or Dijon mustard on the side for dipping.

7. Prosciutto-Wrapped Asparagus Spears

Ingredients:

- 12 asparagus spears, tough ends trimmed
- 6 slices prosciutto, cut in half lengthwise
- Olive oil (for drizzling)
- Black pepper (optional, for seasoning)

Instructions:

1. Set the oven temperature to 400°F, or 200°C.
2. Starting at the bottom and working your way up to the top, encircle each asparagus spear with a half-slice of prosciutto. Continue wrapping asparagus spears until they are all done.
3. Make sure the asparagus spears wrapped in prosciutto are arranged in a single layer on a baking sheet covered with parchment paper.
4. Gently brush the asparagus with olive oil that has been wrapped. Add a dash of black pepper for more flavor if desired.
5. After preheating the oven, place the baking sheet inside and bake for 10 to 12 minutes, or until the asparagus is soft but still somewhat crunchy and the prosciutto is crispy.
6. Take the asparagus spears wrapped in prosciutto out of the oven. After moving them to a dish, serve them hot.

8. Zesty Beef Jerky

Ingredients:

- 1 pound beef (sirloin, flank steak, or any lean cut suitable for jerky)
- 1/4 cup soy sauce or coconut aminos (for a gluten-free option)

- 2 tablespoons Worcestershire sauce
- 2 tablespoons apple cider vinegar
- 1 tablespoon hot sauce (adjust according to preference)
- 1 teaspoon garlic powder
- 1 teaspoon onion powder
- 1 teaspoon smoked paprika
- 1/2 teaspoon black pepper
- Optional: Pinch of cayenne pepper for added heat

Instructions:

1. Cut the beef into thin, 1/4-inch-thick strips against the grain.
2. Combine the apple cider vinegar, hot sauce, smoked paprika, garlic powder, onion powder, soy sauce or coconut aminos, black pepper, and cayenne pepper, if using, in a bowl. Blend the ingredients for the marinade well.
3. Transfer the cut beef strips to a shallow plate or a resealable plastic bag. Make sure every strip of beef is equally covered with marinade as you pour it over it. For best taste, marinate in the refrigerator for at least 4 hours or overnight, covered or sealed in a bag.
4. Set the dehydrator's temperature to the minimum recommended by the manufacturer, or preheat your oven to 65–75°C (150–170°F).

5. If using the oven, arrange the marinated beef strips on wire racks set on baking sheets or on the trays of the dehydrator. Verify that the strips do not overlap.

6. To dry beef jerky in a dehydrator, according to the manufacturer's directions. Bake the beef strips in the oven for three to four hours, or until the jerky is firm and dry but still chewy. Halfway through the drying period, flip the strips.

7. Allow the Zesty Beef Jerky to cool fully once it has dried. Blot off any extra oil. For up to several weeks, keep the jerky stored in airtight containers or resealable bags.

9. Bacon-Wrapped Asparagus

Ingredients:

- 12 asparagus spears, tough ends trimmed
- 6 slices bacon, cut in half crosswise
- Olive oil (for drizzling, optional)
- Black pepper (optional, for seasoning)

Instructions:

Set the oven temperature to 400°F, or 200°C.

2. Starting from the bottom and working your way up to the tip, wrap a half-slice of bacon around each

asparagus spear. Continue wrapping asparagus spears until they are all done.

3. Make sure the bacon-wrapped asparagus are arranged in a single layer on a baking sheet covered with parchment paper.

4. You may gently sprinkle some olive oil over the wrapped asparagus to give some flavor and crispiness. Add a dash of black pepper for spice, if desired.

5. After preheating the oven, place the baking sheet inside and bake for 20 to 25 minutes, or until the asparagus is soft and the bacon is crispy.

6. Take the asparagus wrapped in bacon out of the oven. After moving them to a dish, serve them hot.

10. Deviled Eggs with a Twist

Ingredients:

- 6 hard-boiled eggs, peeled and halved lengthwise
- 3 tablespoons mayonnaise
- 1 teaspoon Dijon mustard
- 1 teaspoon apple cider vinegar
- 1 tablespoon finely chopped chives
- 1/4 teaspoon paprika
- Salt and pepper to taste
- **Optional:** Crumbled bacon or smoked salmon for garnish

Instructions:

1. Hard-cook the eggs by boiling them, then let them cool in cold water before peeling and slicing them in half lengthwise. After removing the yolks, put them in a basin.

2. Using a fork, mash the egg yolks until smooth. Add the apple cider vinegar, Dijon mustard, mayonnaise, paprika, finely chopped chives, and salt & pepper. Blend until the filling is smooth and evenly distributed.

3. Evenly divide the yolk mixture between the two egg white halves by spooning or piping it in.

4. For an extra twist and taste, you may choose to top each Deviled Egg with a tiny slice of smoked salmon or a sprinkling of crumbled bacon.

5. Before serving, place the Deviled Eggs in the refrigerator for at least 30 minutes to let the flavors meld.

CHAPTER 6

DELICIOUS 7 DAY CARNIVORE DIET MEAL PLAN FOR WOMEN OVER 60

Day 1:

Breakfast: Scrambled eggs cooked in butter with bacon

Ingredients:

- 4 eggs
- 4 slices of bacon
- 2 tablespoons butter
- Salt and pepper to taste

Instructions:

1. Crack the eggs into a bowl and whisk them until well beaten. Season with salt and pepper according to your taste.

2. Heat a frying pan over medium heat and add the bacon slices. Cook until crispy. Remove the bacon from the pan and place it on a paper towel-lined plate to drain excess grease. Crumble or chop the bacon into smaller pieces.

3. In the same pan, reduce the heat to medium-low and add the butter. Let it melt and coat the pan evenly.

4. Pour the beaten eggs into the pan with the melted butter. Let them sit for a few seconds until the edges start to set.

5. Using a spatula, gently push and fold the eggs from the edges toward the center, allowing the uncooked eggs to flow to the exposed pan surface.

6. Continue cooking and folding the eggs until they are mostly set but still slightly creamy. Be careful not to overcook them.

7. Once the eggs are done to your liking, remove the pan from the heat and stir in the crumbled bacon pieces.

8. Serve the scrambled eggs with bacon hot and enjoy!

Lunch: Grilled chicken thighs

Ingredients:
- 4-6 chicken thighs, bone-in and skin-on
- Olive oil

- Salt and pepper (or your preferred seasoning blend)

Instructions:

1. Preheat your grill to medium-high heat.
2. Pat dry the chicken thighs with paper towels to remove excess moisture.
3. Brush the chicken thighs with olive oil on both sides to prevent sticking and promote crispiness.
4. Season the thighs generously with salt and pepper or your preferred seasoning blend.
5. Place the chicken thighs on the preheated grill, skin-side down. Close the grill lid.
6. Grill the chicken thighs for about 6-8 minutes on each side, depending on the thickness, or until the internal temperature reaches 165°F (74°C).
7. Avoid flipping the chicken too frequently to allow for nice grill marks and even cooking.
8. Once cooked through and the skin is crispy, remove the chicken thighs from the grill and let them rest for a few minutes before serving.

Dinner: Baked salmon with a side of grilled mushrooms

Ingredients:

- 2 salmon fillets

- Olive oil
- Salt and pepper
- 8 ounces of mushrooms (any variety), cleaned and sliced
- Garlic powder (optional)
- Fresh herbs (such as thyme or rosemary), chopped (optional)

Instructions:

1. Preheat your oven to 375°F (190°C).
2. Place the salmon fillets on a baking sheet lined with parchment paper or lightly greased.
3. Drizzle olive oil over the salmon and season both sides with salt and pepper to taste.
4. If desired, sprinkle a bit of garlic powder over the salmon for extra flavor.
5. Bake the salmon in the preheated oven for about 12-15 minutes, or until the salmon is cooked through and easily flakes with a fork.
6. While the salmon is baking, prepare the grilled mushrooms. Heat a grill pan or skillet over medium-high heat.
7. Toss the sliced mushrooms in a bowl with olive oil, salt, and pepper. You can also add chopped fresh herbs like thyme or rosemary for added flavor if desired.
8. Place the seasoned mushrooms onto the heated grill pan or skillet and cook for about 5-7 minutes,

stirring occasionally, until they are tender and have nice grill marks.

9. Once the salmon is done baking, remove it from the oven and let it rest for a couple of minutes.

10. Serve the baked salmon with a side of the grilled mushrooms.

Day 2:

Breakfast: Omelette with cheese, ham, and sausage

Ingredients:

- 3 eggs
- 1/4 cup shredded cheese (cheddar, mozzarella, or your choice)
- 2-3 slices of ham, chopped
- 2-3 cooked sausages, chopped
- Salt and pepper to taste
- 1 tablespoon butter or cooking oil

Instructions:

1. Crack the eggs into a bowl and whisk them until well beaten. Season with salt and pepper according to your taste.

2. Heat a non-stick skillet over medium heat and add the butter or cooking oil.

3. Once the skillet is hot, pour the beaten eggs into the pan, ensuring they spread evenly across the surface.

4. Let the eggs cook for a minute or until the edges start to set.

5. Sprinkle the shredded cheese evenly over the cooking eggs.

6. Add the chopped ham and sausage on one half of the omelette.

7. Using a spatula, carefully fold the other half of the omelette over the filling, creating a half-moon shape.

8. Cook for another minute or until the cheese melts and the omelette is cooked to your desired level of doneness.

9. Gently slide the omelette onto a plate and serve hot.

Lunch: Beef steak strips

Ingredients:

- 1 pound beef sirloin or flank steak, thinly sliced into strips
- 2 tablespoons soy sauce or tamari for a gluten-free option
- 1 tablespoon olive oil or vegetable oil

- 2 cloves garlic, minced
- 1 teaspoon Worcestershire sauce
- Salt and black pepper to taste
- Optional: Fresh herbs (such as thyme or rosemary) for added flavor

Instructions:

1. In a bowl, combine the soy sauce, olive oil, minced garlic, Worcestershire sauce, salt, and black pepper. If desired, add fresh herbs for additional flavor.

2. Add the sliced beef to the marinade, ensuring each strip is well-coated. Let it marinate for at least 15-30 minutes, or longer for enhanced flavor.

3. Heat a skillet or frying pan over medium-high heat.

4. Once the pan is hot, add the marinated beef strips. Cook for 2-3 minutes per side or until they reach your preferred level of doneness.

5. Use tongs to turn the strips and ensure even cooking. The goal is to achieve a nice sear on the outside while keeping the inside tender.

6. Once cooked, remove the beef steak strips from the pan and let them rest for a couple of minutes.

7. Serve the steak strips on a plate and optionally garnish with additional fresh herbs.

Dinner: Grilled lamb chops

Ingredients:

- 8 lamb loin chops or rib chops
- 2-3 cloves garlic, minced
- 2 tablespoons olive oil
- 1 tablespoon fresh rosemary, chopped (or 1 teaspoon dried rosemary)
- Salt and black pepper to taste

Instructions:

1. Preheat your grill to medium-high heat.
2. In a bowl, combine the minced garlic, olive oil, chopped rosemary, salt, and black pepper.
3. Pat dry the lamb chops with paper towels and brush them with the prepared marinade, ensuring each chop is well-coated. Let them marinate for at least 15-30 minutes at room temperature.
4. Once the grill is hot, place the lamb chops on the grill.
5. Grill the lamb chops for about 3-4 minutes on each side for medium-rare doneness, adjusting the time based on your preferred level of doneness.
6. Use tongs to flip the chops only once during grilling to get those beautiful grill marks.
7. Remove the lamb chops from the grill and let them rest for a few minutes before serving.

Day 3:

- **Breakfast: Sausages with fried eggs**

Ingredients:

- 4 sausages (any variety you prefer)
- 4 eggs
- 1-2 tablespoons cooking oil or butter
- Salt and pepper to taste

Instructions:

1. Heat a skillet or frying pan over medium heat.
2. Add the sausages to the skillet and cook them, turning occasionally, until they are browned and cooked through. Cooking time will vary based on the type and thickness of the sausages.
3. While the sausages are cooking, crack the eggs into a bowl without breaking the yolks.
4. Heat another skillet or frying pan over medium heat and add cooking oil or butter.
5. Once the oil or butter is hot, carefully add the eggs to the skillet, being careful not to break the yolks. Season the eggs with salt and pepper to taste.
6. Fry the eggs until the whites are set and the edges are slightly crispy. You can cover the pan for a

minute or so to help cook the tops of the eggs if desired.

7. Once the sausages are cooked and the eggs are fried to your liking, remove them from the heat.

Lunch: Turkey breast slices

Ingredients:

- 1 pound turkey breast slices
- 2 tablespoons olive oil or butter
- Salt, pepper, and any desired seasonings (such as garlic powder, paprika, or herbs)

Instructions:

1. Pat dry the turkey breast slices with paper towels and season them generously with salt, pepper, and any additional seasonings you prefer.

2. Heat a skillet or frying pan over medium-high heat and add the olive oil or butter.

3. Once the skillet is hot, add the seasoned turkey breast slices to the pan in a single layer. You may need to cook them in batches depending on the size of your pan.

4. Cook the turkey slices for about 3-4 minutes on each side or until they are cooked through and golden brown on the outside.

5. Use tongs to flip the slices halfway through the cooking process to ensure even cooking.

6. Check the internal temperature of the turkey slices using a meat thermometer to ensure they reach a safe temperature of 165°F (74°C).

7. Once cooked, remove the turkey breast slices from the pan and let them rest for a few minutes before serving.

Dinner: Pan-seared duck breast

Ingredients:

- 2 duck breasts, skin-on
- Salt and pepper
- Optional: Fresh herbs (such as thyme or rosemary)
- Optional: Olive oil or butter for cooking

Instructions:

1. Score the skin of the duck breasts in a crosshatch pattern, being careful not to cut into the flesh. This helps the fat render out during cooking and creates a crispy skin.

2. Season both sides of the duck breasts generously with salt and pepper. You can also add fresh herbs like thyme or rosemary for added flavor if desired.

3. Place the duck breasts in a cold skillet, skin-side down. This allows the fat to render slowly and crisp up the skin.

4. Turn the heat to medium-low and slowly render the fat from the duck breasts. Cook for about 8-10 minutes or until the skin is golden and crispy. Pour off excess fat as needed during cooking.

5. Once the skin is crispy, flip the duck breasts and cook the other side for about 2-3 minutes for medium-rare doneness or longer if desired.

6. Use a meat thermometer to check the internal temperature of the duck breast. For medium-rare, it should be around 130-135°F (54-57°C).

7. Once cooked to your preferred level, remove the duck breasts from the pan and let them rest for a few minutes before slicing.

Day 4:

Breakfast: Salmon cakes with a side of avocado

Ingredients for Salmon Cakes:

- 2 cans (14-16 ounces each) of salmon, drained and flaked (or cooked salmon fillets, flaked)

- 1/2 cup breadcrumbs (or almond flour for a low-carb option)
- 2 green onions, finely chopped
- 1 egg, lightly beaten
- 1 tablespoon Dijon mustard
- 1 tablespoon mayonnaise
- 1 teaspoon lemon juice
- Salt and pepper to taste
- Olive oil for frying

Ingredients for Avocado Side:

- 2 ripe avocados
- Salt and pepper to taste
- Optional: A squeeze of lemon or lime juice for extra flavor

Instructions:

1. In a mixing bowl, combine the flaked salmon, breadcrumbs (or almond flour), chopped green onions, beaten egg, Dijon mustard, mayonnaise, lemon juice, salt, and pepper. Mix until well combined.
2. Form the salmon mixture into patties or cakes of your desired size and thickness.
3. Heat a skillet over medium heat and add a little olive oil.

4. Once the skillet is hot, carefully place the salmon cakes in the skillet and cook for about 3-4 minutes on each side, or until golden brown and heated through.

5. While the salmon cakes are cooking, prepare the avocado side. Cut the avocados in half, remove the pits, and scoop the avocado flesh into a bowl. Mash the avocado with a fork and season with salt, pepper, and a squeeze of lemon or lime juice if desired.

6. Once the salmon cakes are done, remove them from the skillet and serve alongside the mashed avocado.

Lunch: Pork chops

Ingredients:

- 4 pork chops, about 1-inch thick
- Salt and pepper to taste
- 2 tablespoons olive oil or cooking oil of choice
- Optional: Garlic powder, paprika, or your preferred seasoning blend

Instructions:

1. Pat dry the pork chops with paper towels to remove excess moisture. Season both sides of the pork chops generously with salt and pepper. You

can also add additional seasonings like garlic powder, paprika, or a seasoning blend of your choice.

2. Heat a skillet or frying pan over medium-high heat and add the olive oil.

3. Once the skillet is hot, carefully place the seasoned pork chops in the pan. Cook for about 4-5 minutes on each side, depending on the thickness of the chops, or until they reach an internal temperature of 145°F (63°C) for medium doneness.

4. Use tongs to flip the pork chops halfway through the cooking time. This helps to achieve a golden brown crust on both sides.

5. Once the pork chops are cooked to your desired level, remove them from the pan and let them rest for a few minutes before serving.

Dinner: Beef liver cooked in butter

Ingredients:

- 1 pound beef liver, sliced
- 4 tablespoons butter
- Salt and pepper to taste
- Optional: Onion slices or chopped onions for added flavor

Instructions:

1. Rinse the beef liver slices under cold water and pat them dry with paper towels. This step helps remove any excess blood and moisture.

2. Season both sides of the beef liver slices with salt and pepper according to your taste.

3. Heat a skillet or frying pan over medium-high heat and add 2 tablespoons of butter.

4. Once the butter has melted and the pan is hot, add the beef liver slices. If desired, you can also add onion slices or chopped onions to the pan for additional flavor.

5. Cook the beef liver slices for about 2-3 minutes on each side, or until they are cooked through but still tender. Be careful not to overcook the liver, as it can become tough.

6. As the liver cooks, you can add the remaining 2 tablespoons of butter to the pan to enhance its flavor and prevent it from drying out.

7. Once the beef liver slices are cooked to your liking, remove them from the pan and let them rest for a minute before serving.

Day 5:

Breakfast: **Frittata with bacon and cheese**

Ingredients:

- 8 large eggs
- 6 slices of bacon, cooked and chopped
- 1 cup shredded cheese (cheddar, mozzarella, or your favorite cheese)
- 1/4 cup milk or heavy cream
- Salt and pepper to taste
- 2 tablespoons butter or cooking oil

Instructions:

1. Preheat your oven to 350°F (175°C).
2. In a mixing bowl, crack the eggs and whisk them together with milk or heavy cream until well combined. Season the mixture with salt and pepper.
3. Heat an ovenproof skillet (preferably non-stick) over medium heat and add the butter or cooking oil.
4. Once the skillet is hot, add the chopped bacon and cook for a few minutes until it's slightly crispy.
5. Pour the whisked egg mixture into the skillet over the bacon.
6. Sprinkle the shredded cheese evenly over the egg mixture.
7. Let the frittata cook on the stovetop for a couple of minutes, gently lifting the edges with a spatula to let the uncooked eggs flow underneath.
8. Once the edges are set but the center is still slightly runny, transfer the skillet to the preheated oven.

9. Bake the frittata in the oven for about 10-12 minutes or until the eggs are fully set and the top is lightly golden.

10. Carefully remove the skillet from the oven (remember, the handle will be hot!) and let the frittata cool for a few minutes.

11. Slice the frittata into wedges and serve hot. It can be served on its own or with a side salad or toast.

-Lunch: Chicken drumsticks

Ingredients:

- 8 chicken drumsticks
- 2 tablespoons olive oil
- 2 cloves garlic, minced
- 1 teaspoon paprika
- 1 teaspoon dried thyme
- 1 teaspoon dried rosemary
- Salt and pepper to taste
- Optional: Lemon wedges for serving

Instructions:

1. Preheat your oven to 400°F (200°C).

2. Pat dry the chicken drumsticks with paper towels to remove excess moisture.

3. In a bowl, mix together the olive oil, minced garlic, paprika, dried thyme, dried rosemary, salt, and pepper.

4. Rub the chicken drumsticks with the prepared seasoning mixture, ensuring they are coated evenly.

5. Place the seasoned drumsticks on a baking sheet lined with parchment paper or lightly greased.

6. Bake the chicken drumsticks in the preheated oven for about 35-45 minutes, or until they are cooked through and the skin is crispy. The internal temperature of the chicken should reach 165°F (74°C).

7. Halfway through the cooking time, you can turn the drumsticks over to ensure even cooking and crispiness.

8. Once the chicken drumsticks are done, remove them from the oven and let them rest for a few minutes before serving.

9. Serve the chicken drumsticks hot with lemon wedges if desired.

Dinner: Grilled shrimp skewers

Ingredients:

- 1 pound large shrimp, peeled and deveined
- 2 tablespoons olive oil
- 2 cloves garlic, minced
- 1 teaspoon paprika

- 1 teaspoon dried oregano
- 1/2 teaspoon cumin
- Salt and pepper to taste
- Wooden or metal skewers (if using wooden skewers, soak them in water for 30 minutes to prevent burning)

Instructions:

1. If using wooden skewers, soak them in water for about 30 minutes to prevent them from burning on the grill.
2. In a bowl, mix together the olive oil, minced garlic, paprika, dried oregano, cumin, salt, and pepper to create the marinade.
3. Pat dry the peeled and deveined shrimp with paper towels to remove excess moisture.
4. Add the shrimp to the marinade, ensuring they are well-coated. Let them marinate in the refrigerator for about 15-20 minutes to absorb the flavors.
5. Preheat your grill to medium-high heat.
6. Thread the marinated shrimp onto the skewers, dividing them evenly.
7. Place the shrimp skewers on the preheated grill and cook for about 2-3 minutes per side, or until they turn pink and opaque. Avoid overcooking the shrimp to prevent them from becoming rubbery.

8. Once the shrimp are cooked through, remove the skewers from the grill.

Day 6:

Breakfast: Steak and eggs

Ingredients:

- 2 beef steaks (sirloin, ribeye, or your preferred cut)
- 4 eggs
- 2 tablespoons butter
- Salt and pepper to taste
- Optional: Fresh herbs or steak seasoning for extra flavor

Instructions:

1. Season the beef steaks generously with salt and pepper on both sides. You can also add additional seasoning or herbs of your choice for added flavor.
2. Heat a skillet or frying pan over medium-high heat.
3. Once the skillet is hot, add the beef steaks. Cook the steaks for about 3-4 minutes on each side for

medium-rare doneness, adjusting the time based on your preferred level of doneness.

4. Use tongs to flip the steaks and ensure they cook evenly on both sides. For a nice sear, avoid moving the steaks too much while cooking.

5. Once the steaks are cooked to your liking, remove them from the pan and let them rest for a few minutes before serving. This allows the juices to redistribute and keeps the steaks juicy.

6. In the same skillet or a separate one, melt the butter over medium heat.

7. Crack the eggs into the skillet and cook them sunny-side-up, over-easy, or to your preferred style.

8. Season the eggs with a sprinkle of salt and pepper.

Lunch: Ground beef patties with cheese

Ingredients:

- 1 pound ground beef (preferably 80/20 or 85/15 for juicier patties)
- Salt and pepper to taste
- 4 slices of cheese (cheddar, American, Swiss, or your favorite cheese)
- Optional: Seasonings like garlic powder, onion powder, paprika, or Worcestershire sauce for added flavor

Instructions:

1. Preheat a grill or a skillet over medium-high heat.
2. In a mixing bowl, season the ground beef with salt, pepper, and any additional seasonings or sauces you prefer. Mix gently to combine, being careful not to overwork the meat.
3. Divide the seasoned ground beef into four equal portions and shape them into round patties, ensuring they are slightly larger than the size of the cheese slices.
4. If using a grill, place the beef patties directly on the grill grates. If using a skillet, add a small amount of oil to prevent sticking.
5. Cook the beef patties for about 3-4 minutes on each side, or until they reach your desired level of doneness. For medium-rare, aim for an internal temperature of about 145°F (63°C).
6. Just before the beef patties are cooked to your liking, place a slice of cheese on each patty and allow it to melt for the last minute of cooking, covering the grill or skillet if possible to help the cheese melt evenly.
7. Once the cheese has melted, remove the beef patties from the grill or skillet.

Dinner: Roasted chicken

Ingredients:

- 1 whole chicken (about 3-4 pounds)
- 2 tablespoons softened butter or olive oil
- Salt and pepper to taste
- Optional: Herbs (such as thyme, rosemary, or sage), garlic powder, paprika, or lemon wedges for extra flavor

Instructions:

1. Preheat your oven to 375°F (190°C).
2. Remove the giblets from inside the chicken cavity and pat the chicken dry with paper towels.
3. Rub the softened butter or olive oil all over the chicken, including under the skin and on top of the skin. This helps to ensure a crispy and flavorful skin.
4. Season the chicken generously with salt and pepper, both inside the cavity and on the outside. If using additional herbs or spices, sprinkle them over the chicken.
5. Optional: Stuff the chicken cavity with lemon wedges, garlic cloves, or fresh herbs for added flavor.
6. Place the seasoned chicken on a roasting pan or baking dish, breast-side up.
7. Roast the chicken in the preheated oven for about 1 hour and 15 minutes to 1 hour and 30 minutes, or until the internal temperature reaches 165°F (74°C)

in the thickest part of the thigh and the juices run clear. Cooking times may vary based on the size of the chicken.

8. Halfway through the cooking time, you can baste the chicken with pan drippings or additional melted butter or olive oil for added moisture and flavor.

9. Once the chicken is cooked through and has a golden-brown crispy skin, remove it from the oven and let it rest for about 10-15 minutes before carving.

Day 7:

Breakfast: Ham and cheese roll-ups

Ingredients:

- Slices of ham (thinly sliced)
- Slices of cheese (cheddar, Swiss, or your preferred cheese)
- Mustard or cream cheese (optional)
- Toothpicks or skewers

Instructions:

1. Lay out the slices of ham on a clean surface.

2. If desired, spread a thin layer of mustard or cream cheese over the ham slices for added flavor.

3. Place a slice of cheese on top of each ham slice.

4. Starting from one end, tightly roll up the ham and cheese together to create a roll-up.

5. Secure each roll-up with a toothpick or skewer to prevent them from unraveling.

Lunch: Pan-seared tuna steak

Ingredients:

- 2 tuna steaks (about 6-8 ounces each), fresh or thawed if frozen
- 2 tablespoons olive oil
- Salt and pepper to taste
- **Optional**: Sesame seeds, soy sauce, or a drizzle of lemon juice for extra flavor

Instructions:

1. Pat dry the tuna steaks with paper towels to remove excess moisture.

2. Season both sides of the tuna steaks generously with salt and pepper.

3. Optional: If using sesame seeds, press them onto the surface of the tuna steaks to create a crust.

4. Heat a skillet or frying pan over high heat. Add the olive oil and heat it until it shimmers but is not smoking.

5. Carefully place the tuna steaks in the hot skillet. Sear the steaks for about 1-2 minutes on each side for rare to medium-rare doneness. Adjust the cooking time based on your preferred level of doneness and the thickness of the steaks.

6. Use tongs to carefully flip the tuna steaks. Be careful not to overcook them, as tuna can become dry when overcooked.

7. Once done, remove the tuna steaks from the skillet and let them rest for a couple of minutes.

Dinner: Lamb stew cooked with herbs

Ingredients:

- 2 pounds lamb stew meat, cubed
- 2 tablespoons olive oil
- 1 onion, diced
- 2-3 cloves garlic, minced
- 3-4 carrots, peeled and chopped
- 2-3 potatoes, peeled and diced
- 4 cups beef or lamb broth
- 1 teaspoon dried thyme
- 1 teaspoon dried rosemary
- 1 bay leaf
- Salt and pepper to taste

- Fresh parsley for garnish (optional)

Instructions:

1. Heat olive oil in a large pot or Dutch oven over medium-high heat.
2. Add the cubed lamb stew meat to the pot and brown it on all sides. Remove the browned meat from the pot and set it aside.
3. In the same pot, add diced onion and minced garlic. Sauté for a few minutes until the onions are translucent and fragrant.
4. Add the browned lamb stew meat back into the pot.
5. Pour in the beef or lamb broth, enough to cover the meat.
6. Add chopped carrots and diced potatoes to the pot.
7. Stir in dried thyme, dried rosemary, a bay leaf, salt, and pepper for seasoning.
8. Bring the stew to a boil, then reduce the heat to low. Cover the pot and let the stew simmer for 1.5 to 2 hours, or until the meat is tender and the vegetables are cooked to your liking.
9. Check the seasoning and adjust if needed.
10. Once done, remove the bay leaf and discard it.
11. Serve the lamb stew hot, garnished with fresh parsley if desired.

CONCLUSION

This cookbook is designed for women over 60 interested in the Carnivore Diet, focusing on empowering a lifestyle that prioritizes health, energy, and simplicity. The diet focuses on consuming animal based dishes, such as meats, fish, eggs, and dairy products, which provide nourishment for both the body and spirit. This approach eliminates the complications of conventional diets and allows for the enjoyment of nutrient-dense meals.

The cookbook is not just a list of dishes but also a starting point for learning about the benefits of the diet, especially for women over 60. It encourages enjoying the pleasures of eating and feeling full, energetic, and in touch with the body. The variety and depth of meat-based meals, from grilled treats to juicy roasts and steaks are carefully created to satisfy the palate and promote wellbeing.

The journey is about adopting a comprehensive lifestyle, not only in the kitchen but also appreciating the importance of nutrition, enjoying whole foods, and feeling empowered to make decisions about diet and overall health. By finishing the cookbook, you have opened the door to a healthier and more fulfilling life. The spirit of this gastronomic journey will guide you through the journey, ensuring a revitalized feeling of health and energy.

9 798886 964454